CONTENTS

KU-053-500

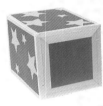
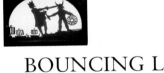
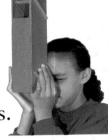
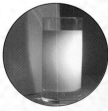

THE WORKSHOP

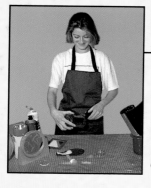

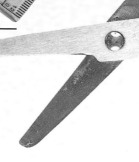

BEFORE YOU START any of the projects, it is important that you learn a few simple rules about the care of your Science Factory.

● Always keep your hands and the work surfaces clean. Dirt can damage results and ruin a project!

● Read the instructions carefully before you start each project.

● Make sure you have all the equipment you need for the projects (see check-list opposite).

● If you haven't got the right piece of equipment, then improvise. For example, a washing-up liquid bottle will do just as well as a plastic drinks bottle.

● Don't worry if you make mistakes. Just start again – patience is very important!

● Now you are ready to start. Turn the page and remember to have fun in your Science Factory!

SCIENCE FACTORY

LIGHT & SIGHT

...ARDS

B48 082 4898   MSC

SCHOOLS LIBRARY SERVICE
MALTBY LIBRARY HEADQUARTERS
HIGH STREET
MALTBY   FEB 2003
ROTHERHAM
S66 8LD

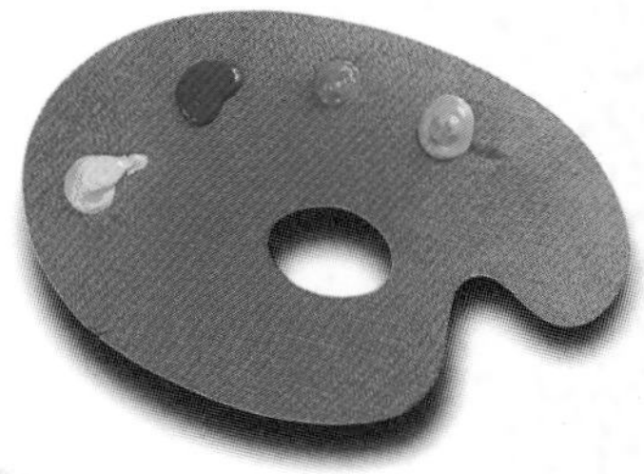

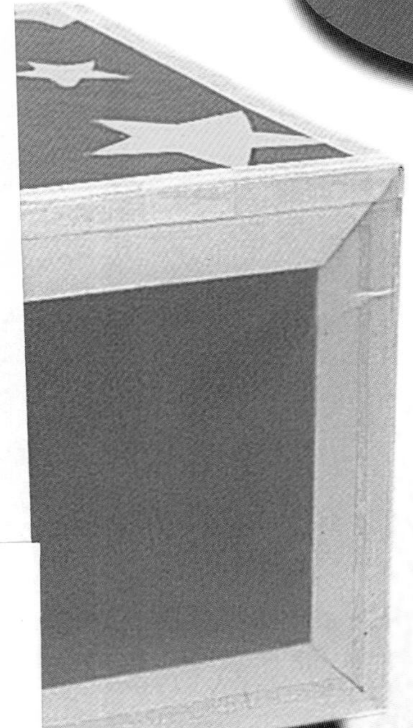

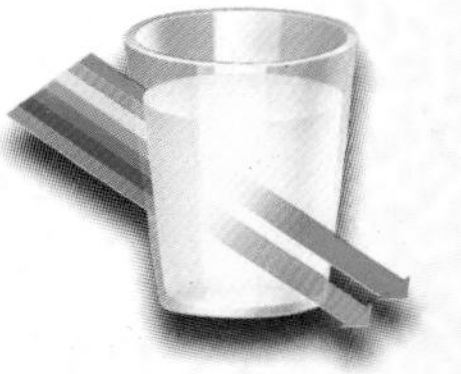

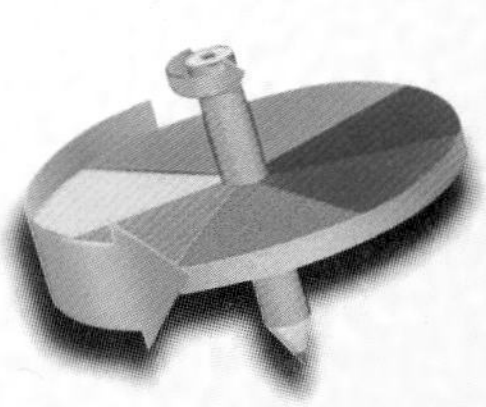

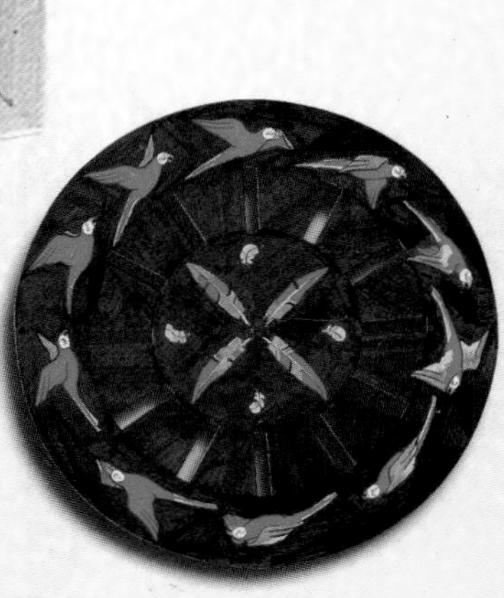

ROTHERHAM LIBRARY & INFORMATION SERVICES

This book must be returned by the date specified at the time of issue
as the DATE DUE FOR RETURN.
The loan may be extended (personally, by post or telephone) for a
further period if the book is not required by another reader, by quoting
the above number / author / title.

LIS7a

FRANKLIN WATTS
LONDON • SYDNEY

© Aladdin Books Ltd 1999

Designed and produced by
Aladdin Books Ltd
28 Percy Street
London W1P 0LD

ISBN 0 7496 3433 2 (hardcover)
ISBN 0 7496 4723 X (paperback)

First published in Great Britain
in 1999 by
Franklin Watts Books
96 Leonard Street
London EC2A 4XD

Design

David West
Children's Book Design

Designer
Flick Killerby

Illustrators
Ian Moores & Ian Thompson

Printed in the U.A.E.

All rights reserved

A CIP catalogue entry for this book is
available from the British Library.

Some of the illustrations in this series
have appeared in previous titles
published by Aladdin Books.

The author, Jon Richards, has written
a number of science and technology
books for children.

The consultant, Steve Parker, has
worked on over 150 books for
children, mainly on a science theme.

All the photos in this book were
taken by Roger Vlitos.

ABOUT THE BOOK

Light and Sight examines the basic aspects of light, as well as its more complex and practical uses. By following the projects carefully, the readers are able to develop their practical skills, while at the same time expanding their scientific knowledge. Other ideas then offer them the chance to explore each aspect further to build up a more comprehensive understanding of the subject.

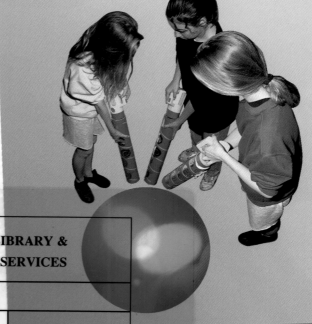

ROTHERHAM LIBRARY &
INFORMATION SERVICES

B48 082489 8

Askews

J535   £6.99

RO COLO927

Equipment check-list:
- Paper and card
- Shallow trays
- Tissue, blotting and tracing paper
- Scissors, sticky tape and glue
- Cotton wool and cress seeds
- Paper fasteners and elastic bands
- Torches and rulers
- Cardboard boxes and tubes
- Modelling clay and beads
- Pencils, felt-tip pens and paints
- Small mirrors and blankets
- Coloured cellophane
- Plastic bottles and corks
- Eyepiece and convex lenses
- Drinking straws
- Large glass bowl
- Clips, pins and nails
- Glass jar
- Milk

WARNING:

Some of the experiments in this book need the help of an adult. Always ask a grown-up to give you a hand when you are using electrical objects or sharp objects, such as scissors.

LIGHT FOR LIFE

WHAT YOU NEED
Shallow tray
Cotton wool
Cress seeds
Card

THE BRIGHTEST AND MOST OBVIOUS SOURCE OF LIGHT IS OUR NEAREST STAR, THE SUN. The Sun supplies us, as well as plants and animals, with light and warmth – without it we would not be able to survive! This experiment offers an introduction to the world of light by showing you just how important sunlight is in keeping plants alive.

GROWING PLANTS

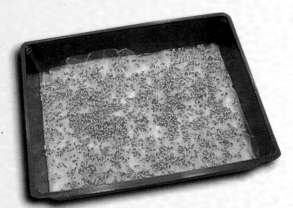

1 *Spread the cotton wool in the tray. Moisten the cotton wool with water and scatter the cress seeds over it. Leave it until the seeds have sprouted.*

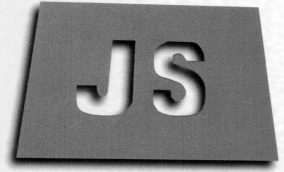

2 *Ask an adult to cut out your initials or a pattern from the sheet of card. Place this over the seedlings.*

3 *Leave the tray in a sunny position for about two weeks, keeping the cotton wool moist with water.*

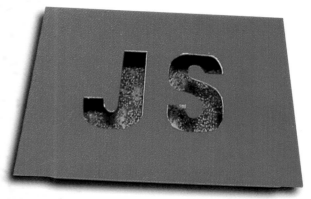

4 *When the cress has fully grown, remove the card. You will see that the cress exposed to the light by your cut-out initials is much greener.*

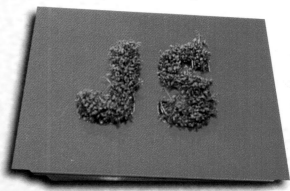

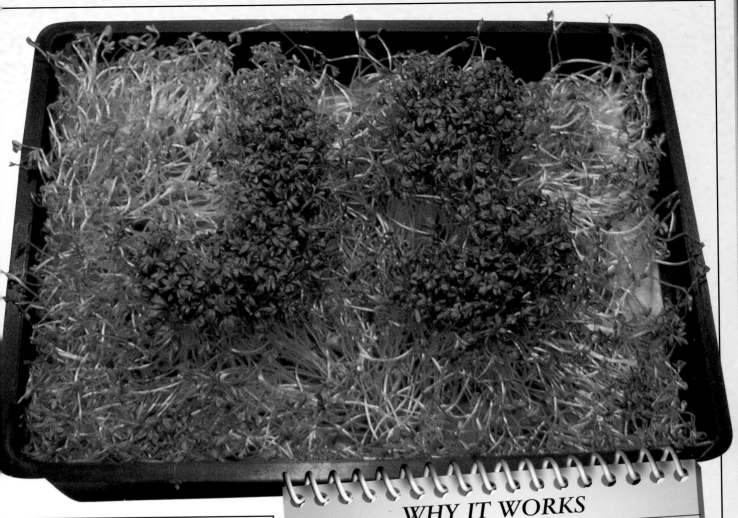

TURNING SEEDS

Plants always grow towards the light. You can see this by placing a seedling on a window ledge. After one week you will see that it has started to grow towards the light. Turn the pot around, and it will start to grow back towards the light.

WHY IT WORKS

Plants use sunlight, along with a gas in the air, called carbon dioxide, and water to make food which they use to grow. At the same time, they release a gas called oxygen into the air. If the plants are kept in the dark, they cannot make their food, so they will wither and be paler than those exposed to the Sun.

SUNLIGHT

CARBON DIOXIDE
ABSORBED

OXYGEN
RELEASED

WATER
ABSORBED

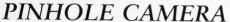

IN CAMERA

LIGHT FROM THE SUN, AS WELL AS ALL OTHER FORMS OF LIGHT, travels in straight lines as light rays. As a result, light cannot naturally turn corners (if you turn to pages 12-13 you will see how light can be made to go around objects). This creates events such as shadows (see pages 10-11). It can even appear to turn the world upside down, as this experiment to make your own pinhole camera reveals.

(if you turn to pages 12-13); (see pages 10-11)

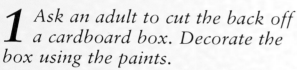

WHAT YOU NEED
Cardboard box
Sharp pencil
Tracing paper
Paints
Sticky tape
Blanket

PINHOLE CAMERA

1 *Ask an adult to cut the back off a cardboard box. Decorate the box using the paints.*

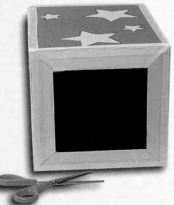

2 *Ask an adult to make a small round hole in the front of the box using a sharp pencil.*

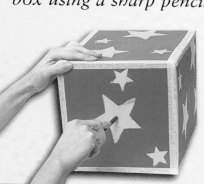

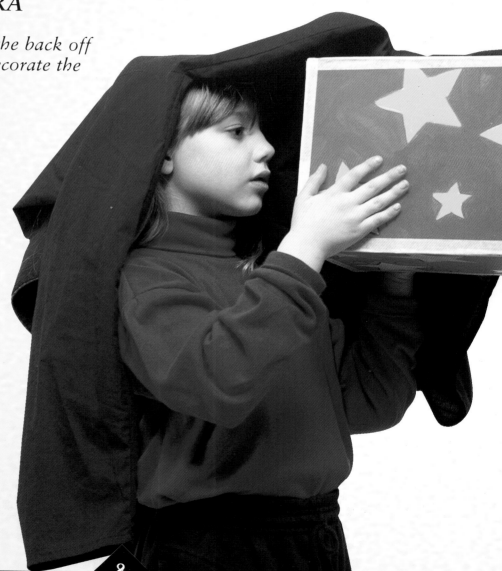

BLURRED IMAGE

Using the sharp pencil, ask an adult to make the hole in your camera slightly larger. As a result, the image on the screen will become more blurred. This is because the larger hole lets more light rays enter the camera. These light rays then hit the screen at lots of different angles, making the picture become fuzzy.

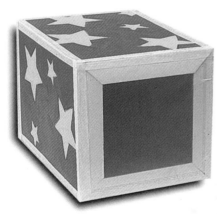

3 Stick a sheet of tracing paper to the back of the box using some sticky tape.

4 Throw the blanket over your head and the back of the camera. Point the camera at a bright window and you will be able to see an upside-down image of the window on the tracing paper at the back of the box.

WHY IT WORKS

The opening of the pinhole camera is very small. When rays of light from the window enter the camera, they cross over because they travel in a straight line. As a result, the image on the screen is upside down. The same thing happens with your eye. Light rays cross over as they pass through the pupil and enter the eyeball. When they hit the retina, they form an upside-down image. This image is sent to the brain, which turns the picture round again, letting you see the world the right way up!

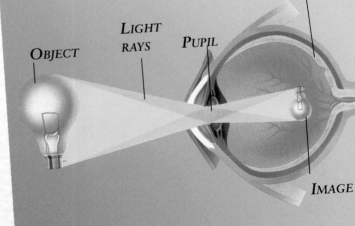

RETINA

LIGHT RAYS

PUPIL

OBJECT

IMAGE

IN THE DARK

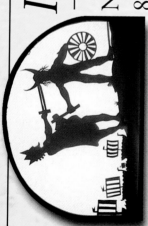

WHAT YOU NEED

Stiff, dark card
Paper fasteners
Tracing paper
Glue
Drinking straws
Powerful torch

NOW YOU KNOW THAT LIGHT RAYS TRAVEL IN STRAIGHT LINES (see pages 8-9), you can explore some of the effects of this. One of these effects is shadows. Look down at your feet and, if it's a sunny day or you're in a bright room, you will see your shadow stretching off in the opposite direction to the light. This shadow is formed because your body blocks out light rays and stops them from lighting up the dark area. Make your own puppet theatre and have some fun experimenting with shadows.

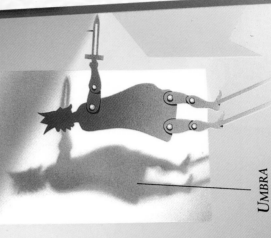

UMBRA

WHY IT WORKS

The dark area, or shadow, is caused by an absence of light. Rays of light from your torch are blocked by your puppet before they can reach the screen. This creates an area of the screen in the shape of your puppet which is darker than the rest of the screen. The completely dark part of the shadow is called the umbra.

SHADOW PUPPETS

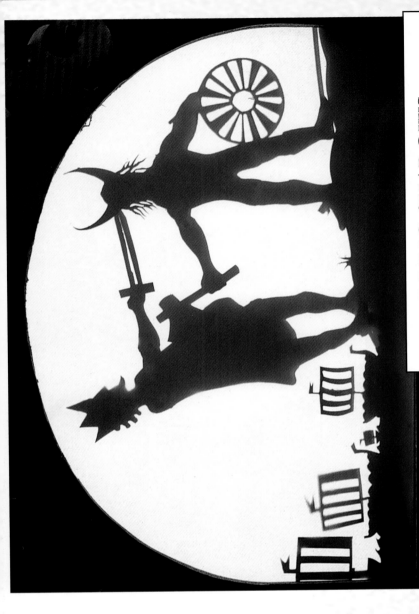

Move the puppets away from the screen and their shadows become blurred, with an area of half-shadow around the edge. This half-shadow is called a penumbra.

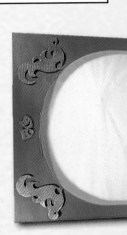

1 Ask an adult to cut out the body parts of the puppets from the dark card, as shown above.

2 Join the body parts together using the paper fasteners, making sure that the limbs can be moved.

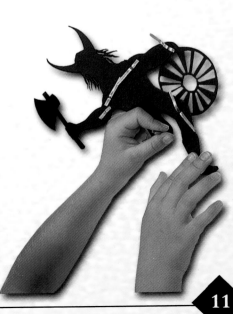

3 Glue the straws to the feet of the puppet. These will help you to control the puppet.

4 Cut a semicircle out of another sheet of card. Stick tracing paper over this hole to make the screen. Stick some card supports to the back to keep the screen upright.

5 Shine the torch from behind the screen and entertain your friends by having your shadow puppets perform a story for them.

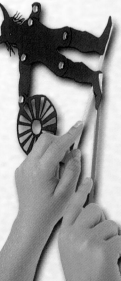

11

BOUNCING LIGHT RAYS

THE PREVIOUS EXPERIMENTS HAVE SHOWN HOW LIGHT RAYS TRAVEL IN STRAIGHT LINES. However, with the right equipment, light rays can be made to go around corners! Shiny surfaces such as mirrors bounce light rays off them. This is called reflection. Use mirrors to build a periscope and see how you can make light turn corners.

WHAT YOU
NEED
Card
Ruler
Pencil
*Two small
mirrors*
Sticky tape

UP PERISCOPE

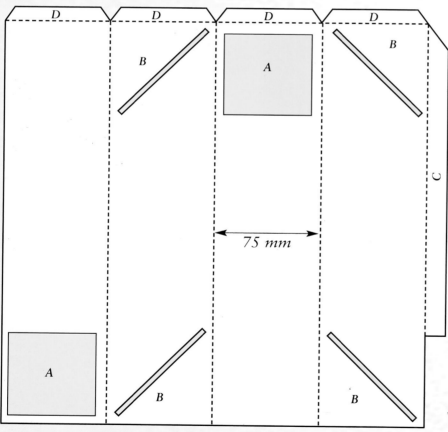

1 Using a ruler and pencil, draw out an open plan of your periscope on the card, like the one shown here. Ask an adult to cut out the plan, as well as two windows (A) and four slits to hold the mirrors (B).

2 Tape the edges of the mirrors. The mirrors should be slightly wider than your periscope.

3 Fold the periscope and stick it together using the sticky tape to hold tab C in place. Stick some card on top of the periscope using tabs D.

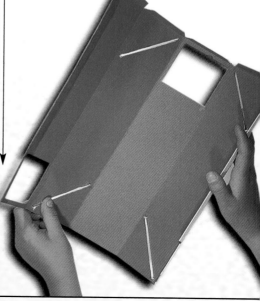

WHY IT WORKS

The shiny surfaces of the mirrors in your periscope reflect light rays. As a result, the rays of light which would normally travel over your head are bounced off the mirrors, down through the periscope and into your eye. This allows you to see over any obstruction.

MIRROR

LIGHT FROM OBJECT

LIGHT REFLECTED OFF MIRROR INTO EYE

ODD REFLECTIONS

Look at your reflections on both sides of a metal spoon. Because the surfaces are curved, they will reflect light rays in different directions, giving you what looks like a funny-shaped face – one of the sides will even turn the image of your face upside down!

4 Slide the mirrors into the slots and use some sticky tape to hold them in place. Now look through the lower mirror and you will be able to use your periscope to see over tall objects such as a fence or a wall.

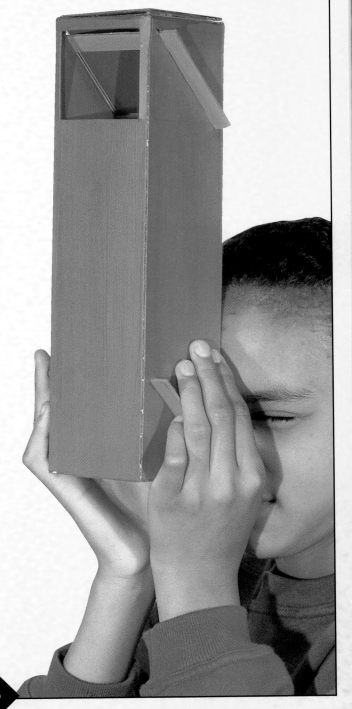

See-through, Cloudy and Opaque

You've already seen how light is blocked by some objects and reflected by others – now you can see how light can actually pass through things! When light passes through something, then that object is called see-through or transparent. However, some objects appear cloudy and only let some light through. They are called translucent. Other objects let no light through and they are called opaque. This project will help you explore things that are transparent, translucent and opaque.

WHAT YOU NEED
Glass jar
Water
Milk
Torch

SEE-THROUGH PAPER

Hold a sheet of white paper up to the light and it appears opaque. Now soak the paper in water, hold it up and you will see that light can pass through it. This is because the water which soaks into the paper helps light to pass through the gaps between the tiny paper fibres.

CLOUDY WATERS

1 *Fill the glass jar with water. Shine a torch through the water-filled jar onto a white screen behind. You will see that white light from the torch travels all the way through the jar and the water.*

WHY IT WORKS

When you pour some milk into the water, the milk particles which float in the liquid scatter some of the colours which make up the white light (see the Splitting Light experiment on pages 20-21), leaving only orange and red to travel through. As a result, the liquid is translucent. When you add more milk, the particles block out the light completely, making the liquid opaque.

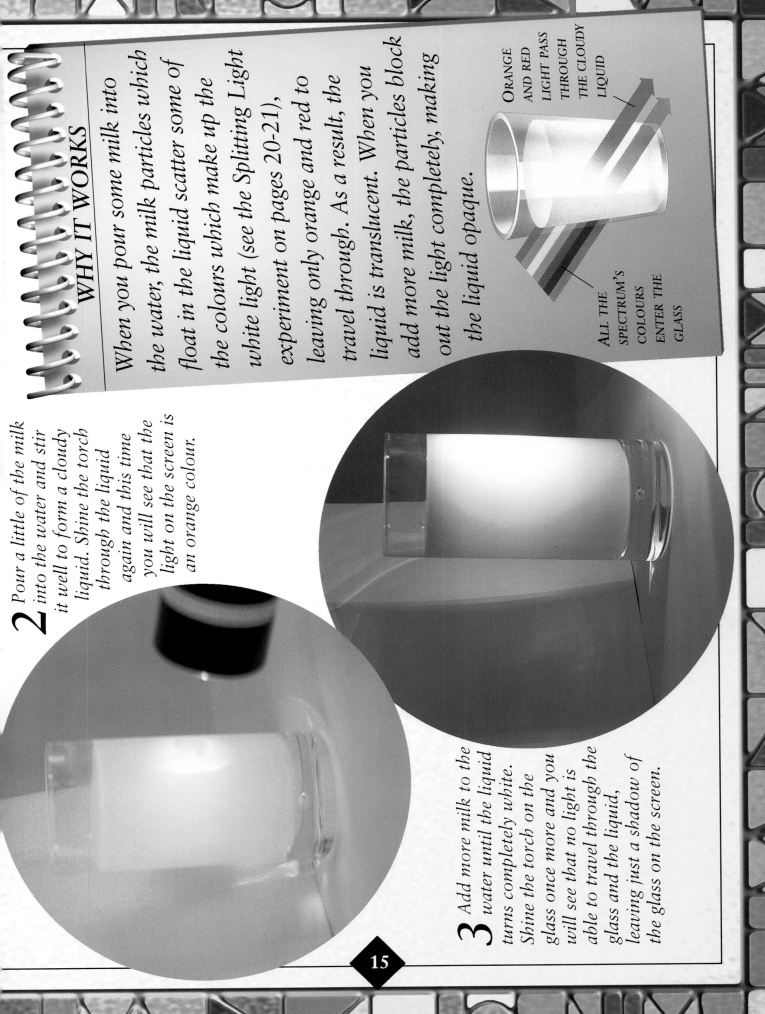

ORANGE AND RED LIGHT PASS THROUGH THE CLOUDY LIQUID

ALL THE SPECTRUM'S COLOURS ENTER THE GLASS

2 Pour a little of the milk into the water and stir it well to form a cloudy liquid. Shine the torch through the liquid again and this time you will see that the light on the screen is an orange colour.

3 Add more milk to the water until the liquid turns completely white. Shine the torch on the glass once more and you will see that no light is able to travel through the glass and the liquid, leaving just a shadow of the glass on the screen.

BENDING LIGHT

THE EXPERIMENT ON PAGES 12-13 showed you how light can be reflected to turn corners, but it can also be helpful to bend light rays slightly. This bending is called refraction. Eyeglasses use refraction to bend rays of light, helping people to see things clearly. Microscopes also bend light rays to make objects appear bigger. Make a simple microscope in this experiment and see how bending light rays can be useful.

WHAT YOU NEED
See-through plastic bottle
Small, flat mirror
Modelling clay
Drop of water
Scissors

BROKEN PENCILS

Fill a glass with water and place a pencil in it. When you look at the pencil from the side it appears as if the part of the pencil in the water has become bent or broken. This is because the water refracts or bends light rays from the pencil, making the underwater part appear as if it is in a slightly different position.

MICROSCOPE

2 *Ask an adult to cut two horizontal slits in the other two sides of the bottle, near the top.*

3 *Push the two ends of one of the plastic strips through these two slits to form a platform.*

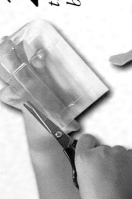
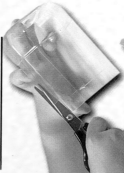
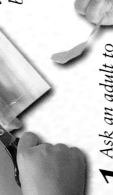

1 *Ask an adult to cut the top off a plastic bottle and then cut a out narrow strip from two opposite sides of the lower half of the bottle.*

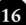

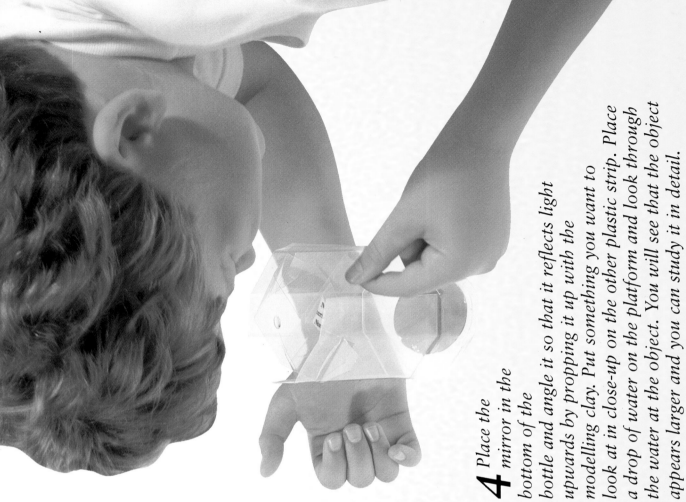

WHY IT WORKS

The drop of water on the platform acts as a small lens. When light rays from the object pass through the drop of water, they are bent, or refracted. This occurs in such a way that they make the object appear larger when you look at it.

4 Place the mirror in the bottom of the bottle and angle it so that it reflects light upwards by propping it up with the modelling clay. Put something you want to look at in close-up on the other plastic strip. Place a drop of water on the platform and look through the water at the object. You will see that the object appears larger and you can study it in detail.

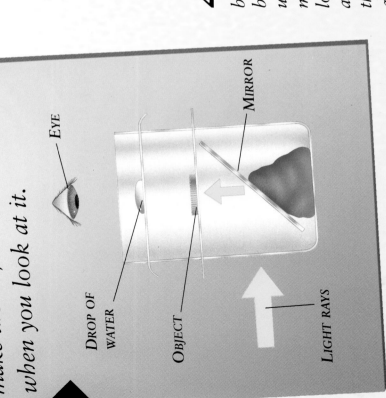

EYE

DROP OF WATER

OBJECT

MIRROR

LIGHT RAYS

BRINGING IT NEARER

TELESCOPES HAVE BEEN USED FOR HUNDREDS OF YEARS to look at far-away objects. Just like the microscope you made on the previous page, many telescopes use bulging, or convex lenses to bend, or refract light rays. This makes objects appear nearer than they actually are. Build your own telescope with this project and see how it can boost your power of vision.

WHAT YOU NEED
One wide cardboard tube
One narrow cardboard tube
Two convex lenses
Eyepiece
Modelling clay

LOOKING INTO THE DISTANCE

1 Fit one of the convex lenses in one end of the wider cardboard tube.

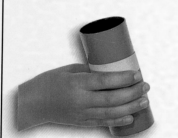

2 Fit the other lens into the eyepiece.

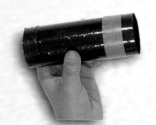

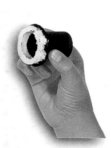

3 Insert the eyepiece into one end of the narrower cardboard tube. Hold it in place using some of the modelling clay.

WHY IT WORKS

The lens at the front of the telescope collects light rays from far away, while the lens in the eyepiece bends these light rays again to produce a larger image. By sliding the tubes backwards and forwards you can make objects at different distances come into focus.

LIGHT RAYS

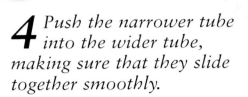

FOCUSSING LIGHT

Hold one of the lenses in front of a torch and shine the torch onto a wall. Now move the lens towards and away from the torch. You will see that the size of the light beam changes as you move the lens. You should be able to focus the light into a small dot on the wall.

4 Push the narrower tube into the wider tube, making sure that they slide together smoothly.

5 Hold your telescope up to your eye and slide the tubes into and out of each other until a distant object comes into focus and appears much closer.

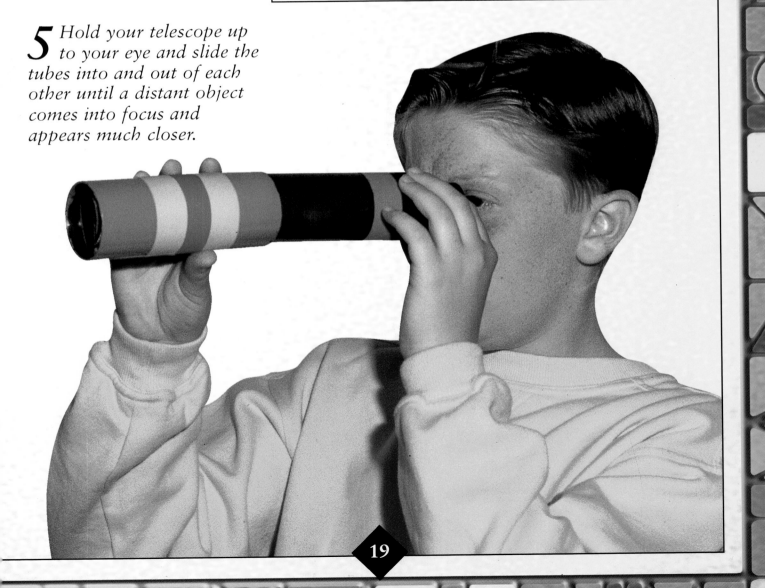

SPLITTING LIGHT

IN THE EXPERIMENT ON PAGES 14-15, you have already seen that light can come in different colours. This is because what we see as white light is actually lots of different colours mixed together. Sometimes these colours split to form a rainbow. This multicoloured band of light is called a spectrum. You can split white light up into a spectrum with this simple project.

WHAT YOU
NEED
*Large glass
bowl*
Clips
Sticky tape
Black card
White card
Mirror

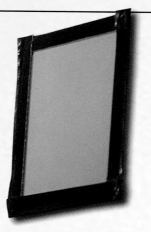

1 *Seal the edges of the mirror with the sticky tape.*

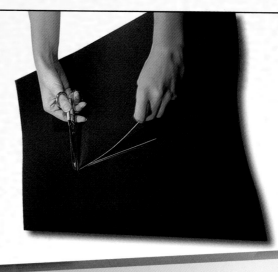

2 *Ask an adult to cut a narrow slit in the middle of the black card.*

WHY IT WORKS

The angled mirror creates a triangular-shaped region near the surface of the water. As This shape is called a prism. As sunlight travels through the prism, the light is split up to form a spectrum. Raindrops act as tiny prisms, splitting sunlight to create rainbows.

WHITE LIGHT HITS WATER

WHITE LIGHT SPLIT INTO A SPECTRUM BY THE WATER

3 Half fill the glass bowl with water.

4 Using the clips, fix the mirror in the bowl of water, so that it rests at an angle.

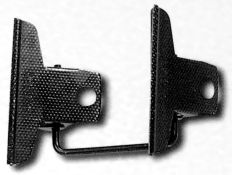

5 Point the mirror at a bright window and place the black card in front of it. Now place the white card below the slit and adjust the mirror until you see a spectrum appear on the piece of white card.

COMPACT COLOURS

Look at the playing surface of a compact disc. The tiny notches etched onto the surface split light up, creating a spectrum which you will be able to see as you view the compact disc from different angles.

MIXING LIGHT

WHAT YOU NEED
Three torches
Red, blue and green cellophane
Three cardboard tubes
Sticky tape
White card

JUST AS YOU CAN SPLIT LIGHT INTO DIFFERENT COLOURS (see pages 20-21), so you can mix coloured lights together. Televisions use this principle to make colour pictures. Look very closely at your television screen (not for too long, though!) and you will see that it is made up of thousands of tiny blue, red and green dots. This experiment shows how you can mix coloured lights to form new colours.

COLOUR WHEELS

Colour a circle of white card with the colours of the spectrum in different segments. Ask an adult to push a sharp pencil through the middle. Then spin the wheel as fast as you can. The colours on the wheel will appear to blur and mix, making the wheel look white.

COLOURED SPOTS

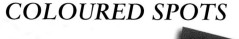

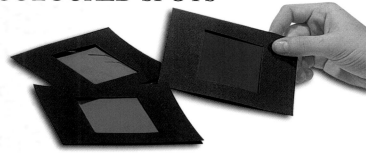

1 *Cut out squares of the red, blue and green cellophane that are big enough to fit over the ends of the cardboard tubes.*

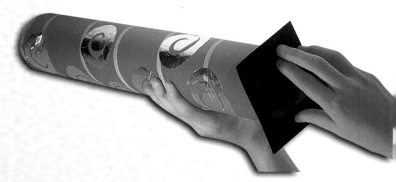

2 *Fix the cellophane to the ends of the tubes using the sticky tape.*

22

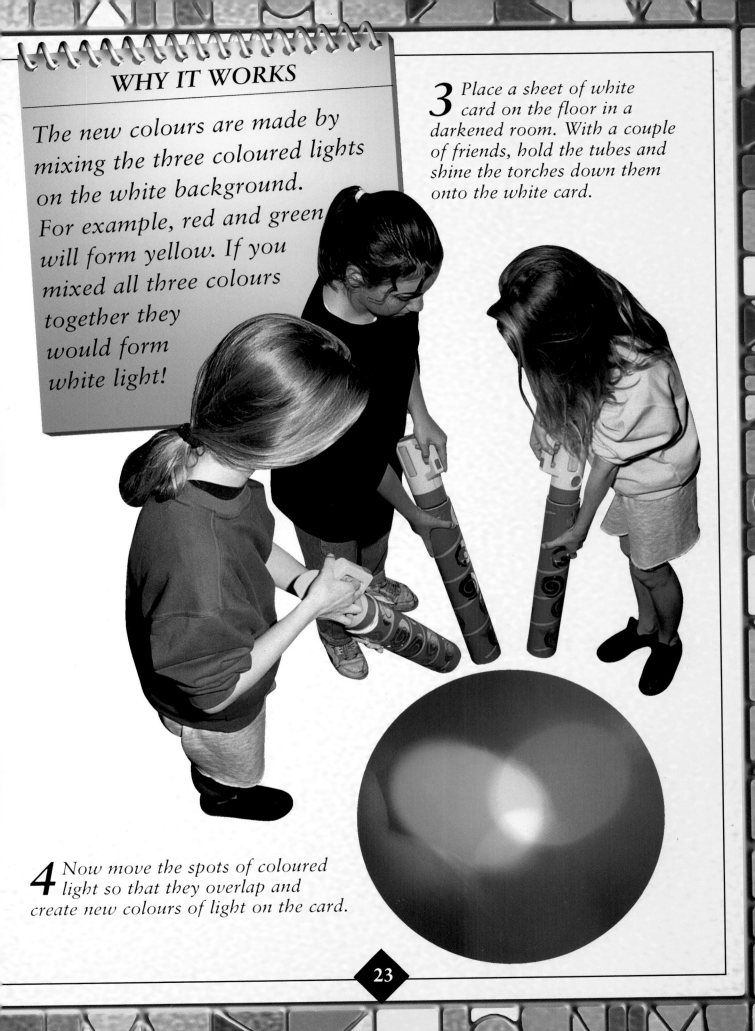

WHY IT WORKS

The new colours are made by mixing the three coloured lights on the white background. For example, red and green will form yellow. If you mixed all three colours together they would form white light!

3 Place a sheet of white card on the floor in a darkened room. With a couple of friends, hold the tubes and shine the torches down them onto the white card.

4 Now move the spots of coloured light so that they overlap and create new colours of light on the card.

23

SEPARATING COLOURS

Mixing coloured lights (see pages 22-23) is not the only way to create new colours. Just like the colours on a television screen, the colours on this book page are made up from tiny dots. Only this time the colours of these dots are magenta (pink), cyan (blue), yellow and black. These colours, called pigments, are mixed together in different quantities to create all of the other colours.

WHAT YOU NEED
*Water-based felt-tip pens
Blotting paper
Bowl of water*

SPLITTING PIGMENTS

1 *Cut the blotting paper into strips and draw patterns on them using a different coloured marker for each strip.*

2 *Place the strips in the bowl so that only their bottom is in the water while the rest hangs over the side.*

3 *Watch as the water soaks up the strips of blotting paper and starts to separate the ink into its different coloured ingredients, or pigments.*

4 *When the water has completely soaked the strips of blotting paper, take them out and closely examine the strips to see which pigments make up each colour.*

INKY RINGS

Cut out a circle of blotting paper. Draw a large spot using a water-based marker in the middle. Then cut a strip from the spot in the centre to the edge and fold it down so that it hangs in the water. As the water soaks into the paper, the colour will separate, forming circles of pigments.

WHY IT WORKS

As the water soaks up the strips of blotting paper, it carries the pigments with it because they are water soluble (i.e. they can mix with water). However, the different pigments which make up the colours are carried by the water at different rates. As a result, the pigments are separated into bands, allowing you to see which pigments make up the colours. For example, red ink is made up of yellow and magenta pigments.

LIVING PICTURES

ALL THROUGH THIS BOOK YOU HAVE SEEN the different aspects of light, from what light is made up of to how light rays can be altered to enlarge or colour things. One other practical use for light is to create moving images, such as the ones you see when you go to the cinema. This experiment will show you how moving pictures "move" and how this is all an illusion!

WHAT YOU NEED
Card
Coloured markers
Nail
Bead
Cork
Mirror

FLYING PARROT

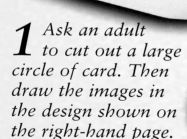

1 *Ask an adult to cut out a large circle of card. Then draw the images in the design shown on the right-hand page.*

2 *Colour in the pictures using the coloured markers. Ask an adult to cut out a series of slits around the middle of the circle using a sharp knife.*

3 *Ask an adult to pierce the centre of the card circle with the nail. Slide the bead onto the nail and then push the cork on to make a handle.*

FLICKER BOOK

Draw each of the parrot illustrations on the corner of a pad of paper. Now flick through the pages very quickly using your thumb. Once again, the parrot appears to move.

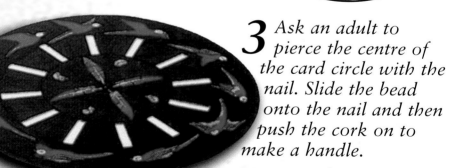

You are not really seeing a moving parrot, but a series of slightly different pictures. When these pictures are seen very quickly, one after the other, they give the impression that the parrot is moving. Cinema projectors work in the same way. They flash separate still images onto a screen very quickly, making it look like the picture is moving when really it isn't!

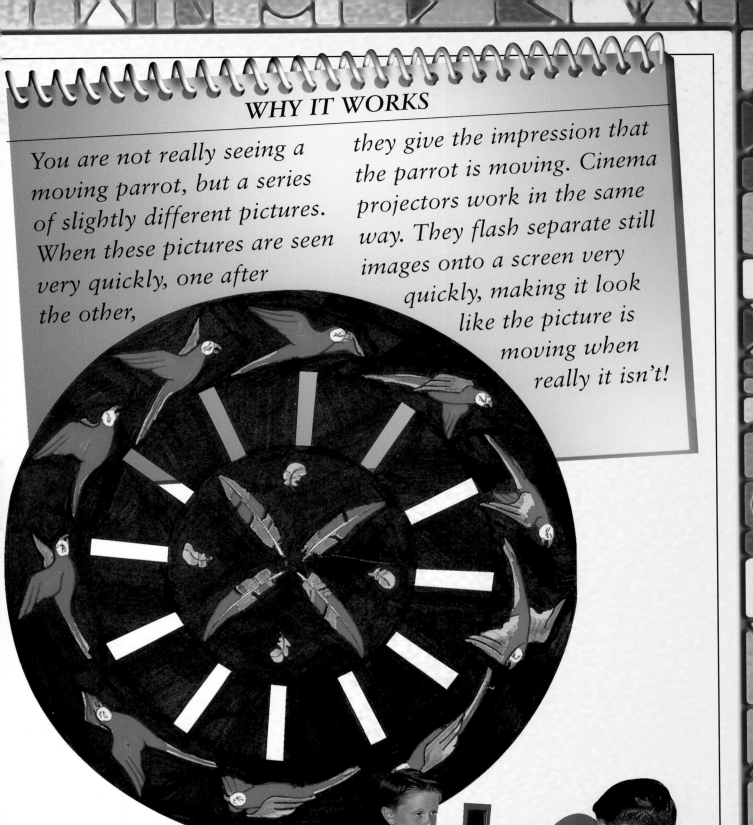

4 Ask a friend to hold the mirror in front of you. Look through the slits from the back of your card disc and spin it quickly. You will see that the parrot looks as if it is flying.

BEAMS OF LIGHT

AS WELL AS PROJECTING MOVING PICTURES ONTO A CINEMA SCREEN (see pages 26-27), light can be used to carry lots of information along miles and miles of special glass wires called fibre optic cables.

These beams of light can carry sound and pictures, such as telephone conversations and television pictures. This experiment shows you how these cables can carry light rays over the bendiest routes, despite the fact that light travels in a straight line.

WHAT YOU
NEED
Black paint
Torch
Pin
*Large glass
bowl*
*Clear plastic
bottle*

FIBRE OPTICS

1 *Ask an adult to cut the top off the plastic bottle. Paint the outside of the bottle black, leaving a small area clear on one side. Using the pin, make a small hole in the bottle on the opposite side from the clear area.*

WHY IT WORKS

The stream of water acts like a fibre optic wire. As the rays of light travel down the stream, they bounce, or reflect, off the sides, travelling along the stream even as it bends. The rays of light hit the stream's sides at such a shallow angle that they are reflected inside. In the same way, fibre optic cables carry light rays along a bendy path by reflecting them off the sides of the fibres.

GLASS FIBRE

LIGHT RAY

REMOTE CONTROL

Your TV remote control uses invisible beams of light to change channels. Try covering the front of the remote control with your hand. You will find that the remote control will not work because your hand blocks off the light.

2 In a darkened room, stand the bottle against one side of the bowl so that the clear area faces out. Fill the bottle with water and shine the torch through the clear area. Place your finger in the stream of water and you should be able to see a spot of light.

FINDING OUT MORE

OPAQUE When no light can get through an object, it is called opaque. *Find out how to make water opaque on pages 14-15 and see the effects of opaque objects with your shadow theatre on pages 10-11.*

REFLECTION This occurs when light rays bounce off a shiny surface, such as a mirror. *Turn to pages 12-13 and see how reflection can help you use a periscope. Can you find any other examples of reflection? Hint, look on pages 28-29.*

REFRACTION This occurs when light rays are bent when they travel through an object. *See refraction in action on pages 16-17 and 18-19 when you build a microscope and a telescope.*

NIGHTLIGHT

Some animals can make their own light. This is called bioluminescence. Fireflies and glow-worms flash lights in their abdomens to attract a mate.

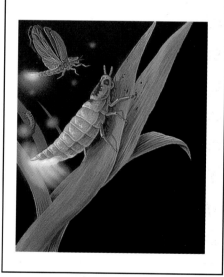

SHADOW A dark area caused by an object blocking out light rays. *Build your own shadow theatre on pages 10-11.*

EYE IN THE SKY

The Hubble Space telescope actually orbits the Earth. It is so powerful that it can see objects 14 billion light years away!

ON DISPLAY

Many animals use colour to display. Birds of Paradise which live in rainforests in Australasia have bright feathers.

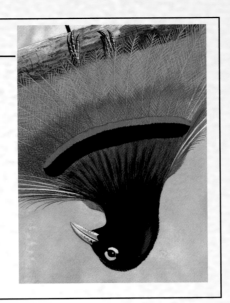

SPECTRUM

Using a specially shaped piece of glass called a prism, sunlight can be split up into a band of colours. This band is called a spectrum. *You can see a spectrum on pages 20-21.*

TRANSLUCENT

When only a few light rays are able to pass through an object, it is called translucent. *See how you can make water translucent by adding a small amount of milk on pages 14-15.*

TRANSPARENT

Objects are transparent when they let light pass through them freely. As a result, you can see through them completely. *Have a look through the book and find some transparent objects. Then see if you can find any more transparent objects around your home.*

LARGE STARS

The night sky is full of stars of different colours, such as red, yellow and blue. Some of these stars are enormous – over 600 times bigger than our Sun!

VEGA

ALDEBARAN

THE SUN

BETELGEUS

INDEX